WORDS APART
Triumphs
over Dyslexia

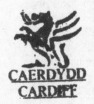

Published by Rily Publications Ltd, 2018
ISBN 978-1-84967-401-0
Copyright © Llinos Dafydd, 2018

The Quick Reads project in Wales is an initiative coordinated by the
Welsh Books Council and supported by the Welsh Government.
Printed and bound by CPI Group (UK) Ltd, Croydon, CR0 4YY

Cover design by Sion Ilar
Cover photo by Lloyd Pursall

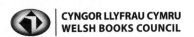

CYNGOR LLYFRAU CYMRU
WELSH BOOKS COUNCIL

Noddir gan
Lywodraeth Cymru
Sponsored by
Welsh Government

WORDS APART

Triumphs over Dyslexia

Four True Stories
Llinos Dafydd

Thank you

I would like to express my gratitude to the many people who helped me through this book, to all those who provided support, talked things over, read, wrote, offered comments, allowed me to quote their remarks and assisted in the editing, proofreading and design.

This book would not have been possible without the immense and invaluable contributions of Lloyd Everitt, Llinos Hallgarth, Aneirin Karadog, Mike Furnham and Catherine Jones who have shared their experiences of living with dyslexia.

I am particularly grateful for the assistance given by Lynda Tunnicliffe, from Rily Publications. Without her guidance and constant help this book would not have seen the light of day.

I would also like to thank Catherine Merriman and Jo Bowers who gave me constructive comments and warm encouragement during the editing process. Also, Sandra Cutler who generously shared her expertise as Chair of Dyslecsia Cymru / Wales Dyslexia.

Lastly, I thank my family: Ifan, my partner, for his patience and support, and for his insightful comments and suggestions; and my daughters Mari, Magw and Jano for their smiles and love.

Llinos Dafydd, author

Introduction

Imagine not being able to read this sentence.

It's not because you're illiterate, but because when you try to pin the words down with your gaze, they dance away across the page. Or the page seems to spin underneath your eyes. The white glare of the paper gives you a throbbing headache. Welcome to the world of someone who has dyslexia.

Dyslexia is not a physical problem with the eyes. It's a neurological difficulty – a reduced ability to process written information. This doesn't affect other visual things. In fact, a person with dyslexia can compensate by developing an excellent memory for pictures. But it can cause problems with reading, writing and spelling.

It's estimated that up to one in every ten people in the UK has some degree of dyslexia. This is a book about some of those people, and how they've overcome their difficulties and succeeded at acting, poetry, teaching and more.

They show that while dyslexia presents challenges on a daily basis, support is available to improve reading and writing skills, and the disadvantages of dyslexia can spur people on to develop creative solutions that give them a different and useful approach to life.

While people with dyslexia sometimes have a hard time

with numbers, time, details, speed, spelling, and too many instructions, many excel at creativity, critical thinking, empathy, entrepreneurial ventures, spatial knowledge and the arts.

What do Judi Dench, Henry Winkler, Keira Knightley, Orlando Bloom, Cher, Jennifer Aniston, Jim Carrey, Tom Cruise, Keanu Reeves and Salma Hayek all have in common? Yes, they're all dyslexic!

One actor who certainly hasn't let dyslexia hold him back in life is Lloyd Everitt. He has invented an ingenious method to help him act – replacing his script with doodles! In the first chapter of this book you'll get to know all about how he deals with dyslexia in his own unique way. And the doodles at the start of each chapter? Well, it's Lloyd's interpretation of the words.

Then we get great input from Llinos Hallgarth, a mum of two from west Wales, who has lived with dyslexia most of her life. She shares things that have helped her along the way, but most importantly she shares the fact that she's always seen dyslexia more as a blessing than a curse. It's all about a positive mental attitude!

In the third chapter we move along to Catherine Jones, who is mother to a dyslexic child, and her struggle in the early days when she battled constantly with the school to get intervention put in place. She shares her frustrations, especially when she, as a parent, knew there was something wrong and nobody seemed to listen.

Then we hear from an award-winning poet, who plays with words all day long! For Aneirin Karadog, it's been about getting to know himself, and learning what his strengths and weaknesses are over time.

Lastly, we have Mike Furnham, a teacher, who spent ten years as a Special Educational Needs Co-ordinator in a secondary school, and has an MA in Special Educational Needs (Specific Learning Difficulties). He shares his take on things, emphasising the fact that while dyslexia won't ever go away, as it's a life-long condition, strategies can be learnt to manage it.

Now sit back, and enjoy the book!

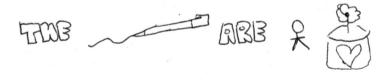

1

"The doodles are my life..."

Lloyd Everitt, actor

I'm Lloyd Everitt. I'm Cardiff-born. I'm an actor. I live with dyslexia. That's my superpower. What's yours?

Not only am I Lloyd, but I've also been known as Jez Andrews, my character on *Casualty* of course, and also Othello. I made history as the youngest actor ever to play Shakespeare's Othello on the Globe Theatre stage – and I think I certainly left my mark with all my doodling, which I will soon talk about. I have my own picture-based language to help me read and learn my scripts – thank goodness for my doodles. Although I'm no Picasso!

I'm a firm believer that if you have dyslexia, you've probably got it for a reason. There's something else going on in your head. Maybe you're more creative in some ways? If you're lacking in something, you'll have gained in other places – that's for sure. It's a matter of finding where these other places are.

Accept it, embrace it.

So there you are. I've said it. And I'm not ashamed of it at all.

Over the years it has affected my mental health. When I couldn't learn my lines properly, it became depressing.

I just feel that dyslexia isn't understood enough. It will affect people in different ways. It's all about getting to the root of how it affects each particular person.

To tell the honest truth, dyslexia feels very different to me these days, almost as if I don't have it. Apart from when I have to read a script that I haven't prepared for.

Some actors turn up and only have to look at a script once, as they have photographic memories. The words are already in there. But I can't read *and* act. I have to *know* the lines. I need to get better with my sight reading, but it's the 'sight' that's the difficult bit. Sometimes, what's down on paper isn't what comes out of my mouth. I mix the words up.

Apart from that, it doesn't feel like I've got dyslexia, because I don't get upset now about not knowing what the words are. The lines go into my head because of the pictures. The doodles are my life now. Whenever I have lines to learn – being an actor, of course, means that there's loads – I draw whatever I have to learn.

For example, if the line is "I've got to go", 'I' will be a stick man, 'got' will be a closed hand, then 'to go' will be the number 2 and a set of traffic lights with the bottom one coloured. The only problem with this system is when I want to draw a word, sometimes there's no actual picture that fits the meaning!

The doodles come from my imagination. They are therapeutic and fun. It makes learning lines an enjoyable experience. You have to make life easier for yourself when you have so many scripts to learn. The doodles I draw are a visual language, like the hieroglyphics used by Egyptians – it's a very similar system using symbols and pictures.

I learnt the whole of *Othello* – and it was a very long process – in around three weeks. But it doesn't matter that it takes a long time because drawing the lines is quite fun and relaxing.

Othello was fantastic. Looking back on it, I'm very proud of myself. I was hard on myself at that time. I'm such a perfectionist.

I had a lot of frustrations in the early days. Sometimes I didn't have time to learn my lines, and I just didn't bother with some parts I was offered because I knew I wouldn't be able to learn the script in time.

I remember clearly one moment that has stuck with me. I had an audition for a part which I didn't get. Then the casting director suddenly stopped reading with me, and I realised that she was crying and getting very upset. She could see my problem.

Although I've had dyslexia all my life, it was only when I was studying at the Royal Welsh College of Music and Drama that I got the diagnosis.

We were doing a section of a play, and I just didn't know my lines. It took me ages to go through the script. I tried to cover it up, and did some recordings. But the words weren't going in and it got me down. Then one of the tutors said "Maybe you have dyslexia". So I took a test, and it was very clear that I did indeed have it.

Looking back, the signs were there, of course. Throughout childhood, I was unable to read properly. In secondary school, when we had to read I would start and go through a couple of pages, but I always had to go back to the beginning afterwards because I had forgotten what I'd read. It wouldn't go in. So reading was a big struggle. But I was really good at writing stories, and that's what got me through my English. I don't come from a family of readers, so I never went home and read to my parents or anything like that.

At school I was more inclined to do football and boxing. I was very sporty. I concentrated too much on the non-academic side of things to notice my poor reading. But it's odd, looking back, that nobody else picked it up. Personally, though, I don't feel let down by the system. But I definitely feel that some children are being let down.

I remember that one of my difficulties was when I had to get up in front of the class. You know, those times when everybody has to get up and read a little section of a book. You know you're not going to read it properly. You're going to try to read it, but it won't come out right. I might swap words around, and then people would laugh.

I feel that from a personal point of view I was able to brush off the laughter. But somebody with a thinner skin could have had their confidence destroyed. It would make them feel unworthy, being laughed at. Bullied.

I'm just thinking of the children I grew up around. Some of them were really intelligent, but came from tough homes. Who knows what their problems and issues were? But teachers just fobbed them off as naughty children. I'm sure, looking back, that there was more to it than that.

All teachers should have basic training in dyslexia. It's baffling to think that teachers might be marking hundreds of English homework stories, for example, not knowing the tell-tale signs. It's a no-brainer that they should be trained to spot something that could cause a child such basic problems. We really do need to catch dyslexia early.

And when a child starts to read and write, it's about staff keeping good records. Just noting problems early and making sure that records move with the child and don't get lost, so the child's progress is tracked through the school. It's about helping the child along.

Of course, you can't force a child to do anything. If somebody had forced me to read more when I was a kid, I don't think it would have improved anything. Reading wasn't something I wanted to do. You have to want to do it, and that's hard as a child. All you want to do is have fun. The trick is to make it fun for children.

In the last year I've been working on short films, on subjects like homelessness and male suicide. It's a new aspect to my work that I really love. I get to write the scripts, and a friend of mine is the director. The writing aspect varies. It's not easy all the time, but that's how it is anyway, even for those who don't have dyslexia.

Somebody might tell you a story, or literally just a sentence, and it might spin your head around, and you're able to write all night. Then there might be a moment when you know that something needs to be changed in a scene, but you're not sure what. So you have to hang in there and wait for inspiration to return.

If somebody were to mark my writing now, they'd say it was terrible, full of spelling mistakes. But dyslexia doesn't hold me back from writing. I'm almost doing the same as when I learn lines. I'm seeing pictures before I write, and then I just free-write as I think.

This is what is so important for you to know. Even if you are dyslexic, any skill can be learnt. Nothing is unreachable. Go for it! That's what I did, and still do.

Work hard at improving it but at the same time, without getting frustrated. Be nice to yourself.

Having dyslexia means your brain is wired in a certain way. If you didn't have dyslexia, you wouldn't have that specialness. Do amazing things, creative things. The world is your oyster. My advice to those who live with dyslexia is to always be gentle on yourself. Don't feel frustrated, or that you are letting yourself down. Negative feelings don't help at all, they hinder. So don't put too much pressure on yourself. Actually, don't put *any* pressure on yourself, just take the steps that you know will help you, however slowly. Write down little goals for yourself and tick them off, one by one. You'll soon find yourself breaking through the barriers.

Self-belief is so important if you have dyslexia. I can't remember anybody telling me to do my pictures. I just had to think of a way to learn my lines, and I was the only one who could help myself. Self-belief is important to everybody who needs to go anywhere in this world. Rewards will come.

When I was nominated for the Best Newcomer prize at the National TV Awards for my role on *Casualty*, that was amazing. My shining moment.

In the meantime, find something you enjoy reading and go for it. I didn't read a proper book until I was about twenty-four. A proper thick book. It was *A Game of*

Thrones. But I enjoyed it, and by the time I'd finished that book, I felt I could read anything. I read more and more as I grow older – I need to. I try to read for half an hour a day. At the beginning I was struggling to get through a couple of pages.

So don't let negative thoughts get in your way when you are trying to read, or to do any tasks that seem difficult. Try not to get frustrated with yourself. Stop kicking yourself. Do anything that makes you relax then get back to the reading, or whatever the task is, when you're in a better mood.

If you have dyslexia and you're reading this, you're on the right track. You've reached the end of the first chapter. Well done!

2

OO SHOULD 🚀 🦷 OF 🙂😊 OO P ✂️ AND ALL ❓

"We should be proud of who we are, warts and all."

– Llinos Hallgarth, a mum of two from west
Wales, who has dyslexia. But it will never
define who she is. Here's her story.

I'm a mum, a complementary therapist, and I work for
a council in mid Wales. Thankfully my jobs mean that I
mostly talk instead of writing.

My main struggle during childhood was school, I
suppose. I had difficulty in primary school with written
work and reading, and was often told off for daydreaming.
Nothing new, maybe, for children – it's quite common,
isn't it? But for me, the daydreaming then often led to
not understanding my school work. I couldn't read to
catch up – so I soon learnt that I had to listen in order
to progress. Due to this problem, I practised a few skills
early on which have stood me in good stead throughout
the years, such as:

1. Memory skills. I practised memory skills and I now have a very good memory. I'm a very visual/auditory learner, and I attribute this to my dyslexia.

In order to improve my memory skills, I used to play a lot of games that involved memorising, such as board games, cards, happy families, 'what's in the shopping basket?' – to name just a few. I also forced myself to read a lot and used to memorise what I read.

I also used to take a snapshot or visual picture of things in my head and use it as a reference, and I still do this now. It must be similar to what they call photographic memory. This snapshot gives me a lot of information and allows me to refer back to it if needed.

A good example of this was when I had a car accident (hit & run) when I lived in America. Due to insurance problems, I had to identify the person who had rear-ended me six months after the incident, via a photo line-up. This was difficult – the person who had run into me was wearing aviator glasses that covered most of his face, plus I'd only seen him in the rear-view mirror. Also, the photos I was asked to look at were of people without glasses.

My solution was to cover the eyes of each face with my thumbs to create the same image that I had in my mind, and to the surprise of the police I was able to correctly identify the person who had run into me.

2. Problem-solving skills. Because I wasn't always able to do things like other children and adults, I often thought of innovative solutions to be able to complete a task. It's hard to say exactly how I do this, but I often don't take questions or problems at face value, and I always think around the issue in order to come up with a solution.

Because of this I know a lot of facts about a lot of things, and I also often get quite obsessed with learning everything I can if I encounter a problem that needs solving.

I am often called 'Mary Poppins' by my friends as I carry so many things around with me in my bag, making me ready for anything. Things like string, scissors, clippers, tape, mixed stationery, dental floss – anything, really, that has come in handy in the past. It's become a bit of a joke that they don't need to worry about bringing anything if they are with me, as nine times out of ten Llinos will have something in her bag that will help!

Personally I'd rather see myself as MacGyver from the TV show as he seems a lot cooler than Mary Poppins, and I often find solutions by adapting everyday things. This habit of mine is something I have also seen in my daughter – she too carries problem-solving tools in her bag!

I tend to think that because of my dyslexia my mental dexterity has developed more than usual or my mind is more flexible, making me a good problem-solver.

3. Stubbornness. If I put my mind to completing a task, I will persevere until I complete it and will try different solutions to succeed. I also enjoy working as part of a team as I realise that sometimes I can't complete everything all by myself.

In fact, I find working as part of a team thrilling. To me, there is nothing more exciting than helping everyone find their skills and potentials, and putting these to work so everyone succeeds. It's a very dynamic, exciting way of working, and everyone wins in my eyes. Teamwork also allows me to concentrate on my strengths rather than my weaknesses, making the result more effective.

As well as being stubborn I am realistic and honest about my skills and abilities. I don't mind making myself do something I am bad at or find difficult, but it is hard. It is easier to be honest about it and team up with people whose skills complement yours, making it a win-win situation.

4. Organisation and logic. Once again I've developed my organisation and logic skills so I can complete work, tasks etc. In order to succeed, I will often have sorted out a specific process to complete the tasks and I have to stick to this in order to get the work done. If this process is interrupted in some way, I often find myself frustrated or unable to do the task as I am unable to see or name a solution to the problem. Some people call this OCD (Obsessive Compulsive Disorder), and I now know that this is also a part of the spectrum of difficulties I have.

If I have a big task to tackle, I have to declutter or clean my working space in order to get my thoughts organised. If I haven't got time to do this, working on the task can be very difficult as everything appears to be too busy and confusing. Therefore, most of the time, I try not to be too messy so as not to upset my mental balance.

If having a 'spring-clean' is not practical or relevant, then lists are my saviour. By listing my tasks, I can bypass the decluttering stage, and tackle the work at hand.

I often have lists upon lists upon lists to help me get stuff done. I also keep a diary, which again helps me organise my life and brain. In my diary I use stickers, different coloured pens, and all sorts of stationery tools to help organise my life and mind. If I were to lose my 'brick' (the name affectionately given to my A5 Filofax by my family and friends, because it is bright red and heavy), it would be very upsetting to me as my life is in those pages. I remember a lot of it as I memorise it. But it is my 'sane' book and does help keep me organised so that my life fits into 'normal', and avoids stress and worry for me.

When I was working through these coping strategies when I was younger, not much was known or acknowledged about conditions like Dyslexia, OCD, Autism, Dyscalculia (difficulty with numbers), Dyspraxia (co-ordination difficulties) etc. I was seen and classed as stupid, difficult to teach, problematic, or awkward as I couldn't do or see things in the same way as other children around me.

I distinctly remember in primary school asking a lot of questions, but often not being given answers I understood, and sometimes not being given an answer at all, as well as being made to feel that my curiosity was a problem. This led to me switching off, which in turn led to daydreaming and not being attentive in class.

Looking back now, I can see that my apparent lack of interest could have given the impression that I was a problem child and stupid, when in fact it was the way I was being taught that was not getting through to me.

When you are in school, the way you are taught does centre a lot around writing and being able to read. But this way of communicating is often quite difficult for a dyslexic person as there does not seem to be logic to these patterns, and I certainly found this the case for me.

Due to this difficulty, you develop and hone a different set of skills, and you therefore get better at picking up other signals such as facial expressions, hand gestures or the meaning of pictures, and your senses of touch, smell, hearing and sight become heightened.

All these are ways of communicating, but it seems that as you grow older, you learn from others that these abilities are not as important or skilful as reading and writing.

I can't remember exactly when I realised that I was 'different'. I think I became more aware of it once people started pointing out habits I had that didn't conform to the 'norm'.

I had been struggling for years with reading and writing, but I was also very clever at avoiding being found out, as I had learnt that if I listened hard enough, I could understand what was being discussed. However, my problems came to a head in Year 6 when it was found that I could not even put a written sentence together, and what I did write was illegible to anyone who tried to read it, so my mother was told by the teachers that I needed additional support to make progress.

I remember her being upset but also understanding, as she too found these things difficult. Despite her own worries, during that year we would diligently go through a spelling book every morning for half an hour. This spelling book moved from very basic words to long difficult words. I think the reason this worked for me is that I learnt these words by rote, like learning times tables. I know now this is a well-used tactic to help dyslexics, it just takes time and perseverance. I learnt a lot in that year, and I suddenly found my literary voice, so to speak.

My first year in the Welsh-medium secondary school found me thrown into an amazing world of knowledge that I suddenly had access to, due to my mother having taken time to help me understand written words. She had done nothing apart from give me time and support to help me digest information, but this had allowed me to learn over and over until I got it right.

I excelled at nearly all subjects, and was offered a full scholarship by Llandovery College. During this time, I thought and was led to believe that I was just a late bloomer, but as the years went on, I still struggled. However, I just got on with it and tried to do the best I could.

It was only when I started doing my Postgraduate Certificate in Education that my dyslexia came to light. I found my first few months of study extremely hard. But I couldn't understand why. I had already done a Diploma in Business, Finance and Media, as well as a Higher Diploma in Business, Finance and Tourism & Recreation Management, so I never thought that doing a PGCE would be a problem – but it was!

So after discussion with my tutor, I decided to pay for a dyslexia test, to resolve any worries I had and to see if it was an issue or not. My day of brain-prodding showed I did have severe dyslexia and a few other issues too, including dyspraxia and a co-ordination disorder.

Suddenly all my niggles, issues, strangeness – whatever name you want to give it – made sense. I suddenly discovered that there were reasons why I was so clumsy. It had nothing to do with a lack of concentration, but was down to a specific condition. Knowing this made me feel more normal.

But I'm afraid I'm still left with a lot of negative memories – many centred on feelings of worthlessness and not being the same as others. A few teachers stand out for both positive and negative reasons.

One very positive example was Cynog Dafis, my English teacher. His encouragement, support and guidance made sure that I excelled in English despite my issues, and I still have a love of the language because of him.

He thankfully did a lot of reading aloud of passages or plays in class, which allowed me to hear the words and digest this information without reading. He also encouraged and expected us to be vocal in his class, which allowed me to grow and flourish and find my voice. Suddenly I could say what I saw and how I saw things, I could express my confusion or question things out loud, and not once did he say my questions were strange or unusual, nor did he ever ask me to 'shut up'. I also remember him saying how much he enjoyed the way I saw different aspects in work that he hadn't seen before.

This finally gave me courage to express myself, and made me feel reasonably normal. However, all this was shaken when I did my Higher Diploma in Swansea, where I suddenly found that all my course work had to be done through the medium of English.

I nearly failed my first year in college. I was told halfway through the year that my written work was appalling, and 'if I didn't pull my socks up, I would be out on my ear'! Thankfully, rather than give up I took it as a challenge, and I buckled down to work to improve my written and verbal skills in English.

I did this in various ways over the three years – I read more, got involved with clubs and groups, and stood for posts such as Student Union representative.

All these improved my confidence and my grasp of English. Involvement with others meant I had to get out of my comfort zone again and develop my reading, writing and verbal communication skills.

It was a very practical way of brushing up on my English language skills, having come from a predominantly Welsh-medium school. What I found I lacked was the subtlety needed in a language. I often missed nuances in the English language, although I was better at this in Welsh. By throwing myself into this English-medium world I found my skills developing, and also my confidence, and I am thankful that I took this practical route to help myself.

I also owe a lot of thanks to my friends for their support when I constantly asked them to explain words that I didn't know that were simple to them. I then progressed to difficult words, allowing me to be more expressive, and to feel that I could communicate much better with people.

Despite sometimes being a barrier to learning, bilingualism in my mind helps us dyslexic people. It exercises the mind, giving us more words to describe or explain what we need to say. I think being bilingual has helped me be more flexible, more aware, and better in logical thought, as well as helping in all kinds of things from day to day.

You can't presume other people's skills, based on their language skills or understanding alone, nor do these reflect the type of person they are. Sadly, though, we are taught that our communication skills do reflect the type of person we are and our status in society. It's very untrue.

I don't like using any of my problems as an excuse, but sadly they can flare up or become an issue when I am stressed, anxious, ill or tired. I get more clumsy – I bump into things, or drop things; I have difficulty reading or writing quickly enough – a short email which should take half an hour to write could take all day; and my OCD can play up so I find myself obsessing about detail, or having to do minor things in a specific order before tackling what really needs to be done.

To be honest though, I've always seen my dyslexia more as a blessing than a curse. It would have been nice if it had been recognised before my late diagnosis, and possibly I could have had more support and reached a higher level academically, personally or professionally.

But maybe not. I will never know.

It helps to know that some of my difficulties are not my fault. This helps me stop blaming myself if I have difficulty doing something, even after sticking at it for a long while. And I have not pursued certain jobs or college courses; the older I get, the harder I find it to change those habits that help me function as a person.

In order to tackle something different or new, I need to be mentally and physically able to learn and have to adapt the way I live my life to reach that goal! In other words, the rewards of the goal always need to far outweigh the stress and hassle it will take for me to reach it.

Despite all these hurdles, I don't normally feel a failure, even if I can be made to feel this when times are tough. It's all about balance for me. So I will always consider carefully before committing to anything, as not completing something is, for me, not an option.

And I do sometimes challenge myself, as I don't want to be stuck in the same place forever. Development for me is so important. Frankly, dyslexic/dyspraxic or not, if you put your mind to it, and commit 100%, you can't go far wrong. There are those out there who will use it as an excuse, but many more who won't, and it is they who need help and support to develop and not let it affect their lives.

Sadly, academically, we dyslexics don't fare too well

at times. Standard measuring systems fail us, as they are not made to measure the efforts of people who deal with information like we do. Standard tests and exams measure our ability to sit tests and exams; they don't really measure our understanding.

I have dyslexia, but this condition will never define who I am. If we are well informed, supported, loved and determined, nothing can hold us back.

It's sad that there's so much stigma around. I think this comes from a lack of understanding of the condition. If people were more open to different learning styles, and encouraged difference rather than conformity, possibly the stigma would not be as bad. We should be proud of who we are, warts and all. We all have issues and conditions, and if we all came out of our closets and shared our experiences, we could inspire other people and hopefully the stigma would fade away.

Knowing that people from all walks of life have this condition, people who are successful, and are managing a fulfilled life, could also make us feel less alone. These people can inspire and motivate children who are only finding out now that they are different, and it will help them to see that they can do anything they put their minds to.

I am a development officer for a language initiative in Ceredigion, as well as a complementary therapist. The way I cope is to get to know my job well. If I can do it very well when I am firing on all cylinders, then if I am ill or am feeling unwell, it doesn't matter so much as I can still do it despite being a bit slower than normal.

The only time work proves difficult for me is if I have to do something unfamiliar, something I am not so confident in, which needs to be done quickly. I find these situations stressful and will often shy away from them.

I wear coloured lenses when I am very tired as reading becomes difficult for me, and the coloured lenses help this. The condition is called scotopic sensitivity, and is associated with dyslexia. The text seems to jump around on the page and the glasses stop this.

I feel that having dyslexia means that I see and interpret information differently from a lot of other people. It also makes me hypersensitive and empathetic to the world around me, allowing me to experience the world in an unusual way. My visual and auditory senses are heightened, as well as touch. Due to these sensitivities, I'm often seen as a bit weird, but thankfully those close to me see my quirks as positives rather than negatives.

I often felt very alone in my early years, very different and very misunderstood. But as I have grown, I've come to see my oddities as positive aspects of who I am, and I love my odd bits!

My whole family has dyslexia to varying degrees. Being

more aware of it has allowed me to see dyslexic traits in my children very early on, and I could therefore get assistance for them from a young age.

There's no shame in having dyslexia. If you think you have it, get tested so you have a rough idea where you are on the spectrum of conditions. If you do, my advice would be:

→ Find your own way of dealing with your own condition. Develop your own mechanisms.

→ Research your condition. This can help you find tools to cope with it.

→ Try not to let other people's ideas of what dyslexia is upset or undermine you.

→ And remember: anything is possible if you work hard at it!

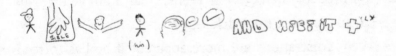

"He truly embraces his dyslexia and uses it positively."

– Catherine Jones, from Blackwood,
mum to dyslexic son, Samuel.

My son, Samuel, is fourteen and it's been eight years since his diagnosis of dyslexia. I had him privately assessed at Dyslexia Org when he was in Year 4 as the school refused to screen for it. We live near Blackwood, and there are no other dyslexic family members.

The main barrier for Sam is with writing. If he has to write, he tends to be slower than his classmates and he can get frustrated with himself when he misses basics like capital letters etc. Day to day he is fine. He can get frustrated from time to time but he generally deals with his condition positively. He also makes fun of himself – not often, but I think that he uses humour as a deflection/coping mechanism when things get on top of him.

When he was younger he could feel snowed under

and would say things like, "I may as well not bother doing this; it'll take me all night and it'll still be wrong". Or "There's no point in doing this; I can't even spell", or "I'll probably be better at French than I am at English; I'm so stupid at English".

His frustrations are more apparent if he has to read large passages of unbroken text. When he reads to me, we tend to select books which are broken up with lots of paragraphs, illustrations and so forth.

Sam also has Irlen Syndrome which means the words can jump around on the page as he reads. This can result in him having symptoms akin to sea sickness. This is obviously unpleasant for him which is why we are careful in our choice of reading material.

When I asked Sam how it feels to have dyslexia, he said, "That's like being asked what is it like to be you." He said he doesn't know what it's like *not* to have dyslexia. He actually talks about it with a sense of pride. But for me, it's a constant worry as to whether I'm doing enough to support him. And I worry whether he might get bullied because his written work is of quite poor quality.

It was a horrendous struggle back in junior school. On the last day of term in Year 3 his teacher approached me and was quite emotional. She said that she felt that she had failed him, but she hadn't. I explained that if she had, I had too.

We had both fought and fought to have him fully screened, but he would repeatedly have just a basic screening from a person from the Authority who insisted that she could find no real issues. The same person re-screened him fully after his dyslexia diagnosis and agreed that her findings now confirmed dyslexia. This was a very awkward situation as I was a teaching assistant in the school at the time.

It was a constant battle with the school to get intervention put in place. They finally put unofficial intervention in place when he was officially diagnosed in Year 4. I was so cross though, because the full measures that were recommended to help him develop and learn were not being implemented.

For example, he was supposed to be positioned close to the board, facing it fully. But when I went into the classroom to fetch something, I saw him sitting at the back of the class with his back to the board. And he was supposed to have spelling work of no more than five common words at a time. But his first set of spellings were ten incredibly difficult words! It was suggested that he have a word bank taped to his desk so he could refer to words to help him. But nothing was done. These were not isolated incidents. This was ongoing.

I was furious. I threatened to remove him and place him in our sister school, at one point. The Head pleaded with me not to remove him and insisted that things would get sorted. But I felt that I was getting nowhere.

Then Sam's teacher in Year 4 who was failing to put in place the required measures was replaced with a supply teacher who took over and did an amazing job with him. He ensured that the suggested measures and learning strategies were implemented immediately, and he also used the teaching assistant in the class to sit with Sam most of the time. Sam's reading progress was fantastic. The teaching assistant spoke to Sam on his own level and Sam really related to him. He came on in leaps and bounds.

Similarly, the Year 5 and Year 6 teachers that Sam had after his diagnosis were superb too. They ensured that his interventions were in place and used regularly, and were completely understanding about his additional needs, which was a huge relief to me after such a long, seemingly endless battle.

His reading now is quite good, and he tends not to struggle with it, but his written work is still quite poor. Sam's main issue is not in retaining what's been taught, but in transferring it to his books.

Luckily, I don't think there is a massive stigma attached to being dyslexic due to the high profile of celebrities known to be dyslexics. Sam says that he suffers no ridicule from anyone at school because of it. I certainly think it's misunderstood and some people still think dyslexics are slow or thick, but I believe the general attitude is understanding.

I spent Dyslexia Awareness Week in October last year raising awareness on my Facebook page by sharing information and facts. It garnered a terrific response from people saying they hadn't fully understood dyslexia. It needs to be talked about and communicated more to the public so that everyone has an understanding of it.

I remember an incident when I was on holiday in Pembrokeshire with both my sons. It was in 2013, so Sam would have been nine. He had a meltdown on Newgale beach because I said it was time to go back to the cottage. When I spoke to him to say his behaviour was unacceptable, he shouted up the beach, "It's because I'm dyslexic". I said it's because you can't have your own way. He tried that excuse a couple of times and then told me he thought it was "worth a shot".

It's important to mention what first made me concerned about Sam back when he was in Year 2. He would be given spellings each week and each night I'd test him, and he would struggle to get maybe two correct. However, on a Friday, he would come out from school with a sticker saying he had scored 100% in his spelling test. I approached the teacher to say I thought he must have been copying because he couldn't get them right with me during the week. But the teacher just said, "He's a boy", and "It depends what mood he's in". It was a battle from then on.

Sadly, it's the norm for people to assume that boys aren't willing to put as much effort into their work as girls. But I know my son, and I know he should be able to write his own name by Year 2! However, I was also assured by the Authority's external assessor that he was a "typical boy".

When you know something is wrong but nobody is listening, it's incredibly frustrating and distressing. Nobody knows a child like his or her parents, so my top tip to parents with children with dyslexia, and especially to parents who think their children may have dyslexia, is FIGHT FIGHT FIGHT.

The secondary school Sam currently attends is fantastic. They have robust help in place for him and ensure that he makes steady and consistent progress. They also ensure that he has extra time in exams and the required resources on hand to help him. The school has been a tremendous support from day one.

You know your child; you need to push to get things sorted for them. Nobody else will. I knew when he was in Year 3 and still couldn't spell his name that he wasn't "being lazy" or "being a typical boy".

I honestly believe that dyslexia is the reason Sam is such a determined and considerate character. He truly embraces his dyslexia and uses it positively. He doesn't dwell on it. He doesn't use it as an excuse (not since the Newgale beach episode!).

He is now an example of how hard work can pay off. He's very good at drawing. He's constantly sketching and he is determined to become a graphic designer. I have no doubt he'll be a very successful one too! Sam is a little soldier. He works so hard and he can't wait to get a part-time job and earn money.

If you met Sam you'd see there are lots of positives with dyslexia. He's always able to find a way around situations. He's a very logical thinker and has fantastic reasoning skills. Dyslexia drives his ambition and his ideas, so although it sounds strange, I'm thankful to dyslexia for that.

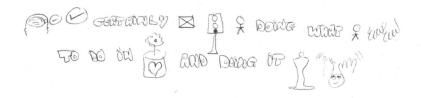

4

"Dyslexia certainly hasn't stopped me doing what I want to do in life, and doing it successfully."

– Aneirin Karadog is an award-winning poet, a writer, a PhD student and a TV presenter. He won the bardic chair at the National Eisteddfod in 2016 and won another award at the Wales Book of the Year ceremony in 2017 for a collection of his poems.

When I got the diagnosis, I was so glad in one sense. I had the test in response to poor academic progress at university. There were two options: either there was something wrong that needed attention or I was just lazy and was going to get kicked off the course.

The confirmation that I was dyslexic meant I could continue to do my degree. But then I suddenly realised that it was a label I would have to carry for the rest of my days. Not the most pleasant realisation.

But I had noticed certain little things that were connected with my dyslexia from an early age, without knowing at the time, of course. Reading novels was hard, and I often had to read sentences again after struggling the first time. When writing, my 't' and 'h' would always be the wrong way round, and I often mixed up letters. I also misread words. Reading quickly, I would assume that I had read a certain word but it would actually be a similar-looking word with a totally different meaning.

I encountered this recently, as I proofread something I wrote about the poet Hedd Wyn, in Welsh. I went over the text a few times before sending it off, and only later realised that I had written about Hedd Wyn's 'clwt' instead of his 'cwlt' (cult)! 'Clwt' in Welsh means a cloth or a nappy!

During my childhood, I was more comfortable reading poetry than novels. There was less going on on the page. It was daunting to see that others could read faster than me.

I've felt a bit down at times about my abilities. But thankfully it hasn't caused any depression or mental health problems. I'm lucky in one sense as I only have mild to moderate dyslexia. It's not as bad as it is for some people, where words are literally jumping on the page.

I don't feel that having dyslexia carries any stigma among my peers. But with the older generation, it's a factor. Many don't understand the condition. There are so many medical and technical terms these days for things that are very real, but which weren't known about many years ago. There's always that problem of generational differences of opinion, with some thinking that dyslexia doesn't really exist.

A computer makes my life much easier. I also used to have coloured cards to help me settle the words on the page, but that felt like I was carrying tools to cope with a handicap, so I haven't used them. I like to pick up and enjoy a book without those cards.

If I need to read I simply allow more time, and I accept that when I'm writing poems, proofreading is very difficult. If I've been commissioned to write a poem to be published in a magazine, and I haven't got time for someone else to look over my work, I try my best to take my time and proofread it several times, in detail, to make sure things are spelled correctly, and that there aren't any typos.

I find it easier to read in Welsh as it's my first language and it's what comes more naturally to me. I speak Breton as well. I've always had languages around me. We spoke Welsh, French and Breton at home.

Fondness for poetry has been there since I was a child. I've been writing poems since I was fifteen years old – it's a real passion of mine. In Year 10 at school I wrote a poem that won me the bardic chair in the school eisteddfod, and, from then on, my interest in writing poetry has progressed. My struggles with words have never got in my way. At the time I didn't even think of the hurdles I had to overcome in my battle with words. But of course, I didn't know that I had dyslexia then, so I just carried on.

There were no special measures at school to help me. But the fact that I didn't get my diagnosis earlier didn't make me think that I shouldn't bother doing this, that or the other, or go in the creative writing direction.

As a *cynganeddwr*, I've managed to write the poetry without too much hassle. *Cynghanedd* is a strict form of Welsh poetry, which has rules relating to the use of rhyme, rhythm and alliteration in order to form a distinctive sound. Once you've learnt the rules, it becomes second nature. The process happens quite quickly when I'm writing and mind-processing.

But sometimes I read something and think it's *cynghanedd* and it's not. It's as if I'm being tricked. In one way, it makes me think in a different way to other *cynganeddwyr*, which is a good thing. Of course, sometimes I can miss the obvious, and it takes a while to come. There might be a pattern of words that should be obvious, but it isn't until later on that I realise I could have done it differently.

I suppose it's like having a sublanguage in my system: it's been learnt, and it's a part of my mind's way of thinking. To me, dyslexia means getting to know yourself, and what measures you need to take to guide yourself in the right direction. I've come to learn what my strengths and weaknesses are over time.

In the past, I've presented TV programmes like *Heno* on S4C. When I have to go in front of a camera I usually don't have the luxury of having autocue. I usually learn the script beforehand, and sometimes I will write a script on location so I have a general idea of what I want to say. Then I'll go ahead and formulate it on the spot. I make good use of my mind and memory. Links in the studio tend to be short, so I don't feel that dyslexia has hindered me in any way.

Dyslexia certainly hasn't stopped me doing what I want to do in life, and doing it successfully. It can be off-putting at times, but there are ways to enjoy literature without reading – by listening to audio books, for example. Technology offers us a way forward.

I feel it's a part of who I am, and in that sense you can actually become proud of what you are and what you've achieved. For those who have dyslexia, it isn't the end of the world, and it certainly doesn't stop you from achieving things even in fields where you would think dyslexia would impair your ability.

Try to explore different techniques and aids that are available and see what works for you. But ultimately, don't let it hold you back. Use it to your advantage. It's nothing to be ashamed of. In the end it's a condition that is a part of you and forms your way of thinking. Don't ever let dyslexia put you off literature or creativity. Don't let it hinder anything you want to achieve in life.

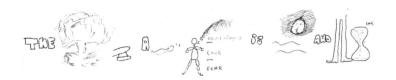

5

"The impact on a child's self-esteem is significant and long-lasting."

– Mike Furnham, a teacher, who spent ten years
as a Special Educational Needs Co-ordinator in
a secondary school, and has an MA in Special
Educational Needs (Specific Learning Difficulties)

It may be a cliché to start off with this famous quote, but it's very relevant to dyslexia:

"Everybody is a genius. But if you judge a fish by its ability to climb a tree, it will live its whole life believing that it is stupid." – Albert Einstein

Dyslexia comes from the Greek: *dys* – difficulty, *lexia* – with words. If you think of reading or spelling as being the ability to decode and/or comprehend a difficult code, then dyslexia is like having the ability to see the code but not having the ability to understand that code. (Think Bletchley Park and the Enigma code.)

The written word either becomes meaningless, or a huge mountain to climb each time you are asked to use it. For a child, school therefore becomes a continual reminder of their inability to do what others find simple and straightforward. The impact on a child's self-esteem is significant and long-lasting.

One of the most common barriers for sufferers is the inability to decode written words and/or to comprehend what they have read. Also, the inability to understand, organise or write down what they have read – "my ideas seem to stop at my elbow, I cannot write it down".

Self-esteem issues are common, of course – limiting a person's ambition and reducing the likelihood that they will reach their academic, social and life potential.

Dyslexia does not go away – it is life-long – but strategies can be learnt to manage it. Over the years, I've learnt a lot about the condition while dealing with a variety of sufferers.

Each dyslexic child is different in their reaction to diagnosis, their desire to overcome the problem, and their willingness to accept that they have to work differently, using strategies they can be taught. The fact is that what works to solve a problem with one child, often will not work with another.

In my research, I've learned that there are many programmes which try to address the specific learning difficulty of dyslexia, but to my mind it is the outlook of the individual supporting the dyslexic that really makes the difference. Being relentlessly positive and seeing the bigger life picture is essential for success.

Recognising and trying to deal with the condition early on in school may be difficult. During their training, student teachers will have at best a two-hour lecture on the full range of Additional Learning Needs, of which dyslexia is only one. There should be a constant top-up of training during a teacher's career, but cost and time demands often make this impossible. The other problem is that a diagnosis still too often comes too late. It's only made when a pupil falls behind his peers, and it can take up to the age of nine to get a clear diagnosis.

Every teacher has a basic knowledge of strategies to help a dyslexic pupil learn, but in the end good quality teaching is what counts – well-structured lessons, key vocabulary introduced and learned, and writing frames to help with extended writing and so on.

To make life a bit easier for dyslexics, relentless positivity is very important – there is no magic wand, but if extra provision is put in place with positive support and strategies are taught, then dyslexics can succeed. Finding and naming dyslexic role models who have succeeded can be very positive.

Over the years, I've seen many coping mechanisms.

Personally, I like the use of mind mapping, which is the use of coloured diagrams of connecting thoughts, often spanning out from a central idea. This can be useful both to record and revise notes. Sticky notes are useful to organise ideas, as is the use of dictaphones to record work or ideas before writing or typing. The only problem with using a computer in the classroom is that it sets children apart from their peers and children do not like to be different.

It's so important for dyslexics to keep going – I'd say to them, seek out your strengths. We all have some. Use these strengths to overcome the difficulties you have. If you cannot write your notes, then use pictures. Find a strategy that works for you and develop it. Find great role models who have succeeded. Have high expectations of yourself – you can achieve! And for those who have to deal with dyslexics day in, day out, relentless positivity is key, along with high expectations.

But most important is TIME to help the person with dyslexia succeed. This helps them to help themselves.

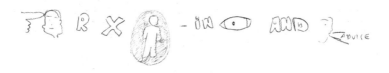

6

You are not alone – insight and advice. How do I know if I or someone else has dyslexia?

Dyslexia is a neurological condition. The brain of a person with dyslexia processes written and spoken information slightly differently.

Not everyone who has dyslexia is aware of it. While you can only be diagnosed with dyslexia by an expert, if you have some of these symptoms it may be a sign that you should seek out an assessment.

The most common sign is that you confuse visually similar words, such as 'cat' and 'cot'. Another sign is that you confuse the name of objects, such as 'table' and 'chair', or struggle to find the right word at all. If you often lose your place when reading, or must re-read paragraphs a few times before you understand them, that can also be a sign. Further indications could include a difficulty differentiating between left and right, having trouble reading a map, or becoming confused when you must follow multiple instructions.

The signs are very similar in children. A delay in learning to speak, or being slow to learn new words, can be a sign of dyslexia. Children with dyslexia will sometimes enjoy being read to but will avoid reading books themselves. A family history of dyslexia is also a strong indicator.

There are also strengths to being dyslexic. A person with dyslexia will often be creative and have a good imagination, and will be quick to grasp new ideas.

The condition of dyslexia is of course a spectrum. All of us have had times when we can't find the right word! Many people are mildly dyslexic and go about their lives without ever getting a diagnosis. But if many of the above symptoms are familiar to you, it may be worth getting further advice.

Helping a person with dyslexia at work or at school

At work or school, it can help a person with dyslexia if they can avoid being given complex instructions. It can also help to give them the instructions verbally and slowly. When you can't avoid giving instructions in text form, make sure they're not very complex. Demonstrating the task you want done yourself can also help the person remember and understand. With children, it can sometimes be difficult to get their full attention, as they may be tired or distracted by other tasks. If that is the case, avoid giving instructions until they are giving you their full attention.

People with dyslexia often prefer to see instructions in pictures rather than in written form. Colour coding can also be helpful for that reason.

Children with dyslexia will sometimes talk to themselves when copying down words and instructions. This helps them remember the information and is to be encouraged. A good memory for spoken instructions can be key to tackling some of the problems associated with having dyslexia.

It's important to recognise that dyslexic children and adults have different strengths and weaknesses, and to be patient. Having dyslexia can cause self-doubt and a lack of self-esteem. Be aware of this and show that you value them and their efforts.

Dyslexic or not, we all remember things more easily if an instruction is given to us in a simple, easy to understand way, and we all respond better to praise and encouragement. So helping people with dyslexia can help us become better at communicating with everyone else, too!

We all have strengths and weaknesses. And people with dyslexia will often have to take their dyslexia into account when choosing a job or career. Choosing a job which is likely to create dyslexia-related difficulties can cause stress, which in turn can lead to stress-related illness. A job as a literary critic or novelist may not be your cup of tea! However, people with dyslexia have been known to thrive in jobs such as sales, art and design, entertainment, acting, engineering, architecture, and computer animation.

It's worth remembering that you are under no obligation to tell an employer that you have dyslexia. However, if a job interview process is likely to involve reading or writing, it may be worth letting them know and giving them an assessment report so they can make adjustments for you.

Dyslexic students at university can also get a lot of help. Most universities have student support, and a specific staff member within each department who helps students with any extra needs. Lecturers and personal tutors will also be told, should you wish, that you are dyslexic and will make plans to help you out. Extra time and the use of a computer during exams can be made available. You will, however, need to present the university with an assessment report showing that you have dyslexia.

Helping a person with dyslexia at home or out and about

Dyslexic children need extra help and encouragement at home, as their time at school will often be more challenging and tiring for them.

If they're losing heart, tell them about some of the people whose stories you've read in this book and how they've succeeded because of, and despite, the challenges people with dyslexia face. Tell them about other famous people beyond Wales who have succeeded with dyslexia: the scientist Albert Einstein, the inventor and artist Leonardo da Vinci, the creator of the iPad Steve Jobs, the artist Pablo Picasso. In fact, many of the most famous and creative people who have ever lived have been dyslexic!

Apart from boosting their self-esteem, there are plenty of ways that you can boost the self-confidence of a person with dyslexia. These involve improving memory, and helping with instructions, spelling and reading.

Memory can be improved by playing memory games. These include matching pictures, or remembering sequences or words that rhyme with each other. For example, play 'I spy with my little eye' to match certain words with certain sounds.

Reading can be very difficult for a child with dyslexia. Words can jump around the page, letters can appear blurred and go in and out of focus, and words can break into two and appear like double vision. This can cause headaches and make it difficult to track words across the page. If your child lacks confidence reading alone, consider reading a page, a paragraph or even a sentence in turn.

Many dyslexic people are sensitive to the glare of a white background on the page, white board or computer screen. Red text on a white background can be particularly challenging. A cream or pastel-coloured background can help, as well as coloured overlays (particularly pink and green) or tinted glasses, which can also stop the words from moving around. The child will also find it easier to read large, wide-spaced print.

Make spelling fun with games such as Scrabble, hangman or a word search. Use mnemonics to aid spelling, such as 'You hear with your ear', or 'A friend is there to the end'. There are many online games that are designed specifically to help children and adults with dyslexia.

You can also practise following instructions at home. To make things fun for the child, turn the tables and ask them to give you instructions. By following them to the letter, even when the child makes a mistake, you can teach them the importance of accurate instructions.

Most children learn to write by forming individual letters first and then joining them up later. Because children with dyslexia are much more likely to remember how to write a word if they develop a physical memory of it, it is easier to stick to what is called 'continuous cursive' from the start. Continuous cursive means writing letters, and then words, in one flowing movement, without raising the pen from the paper.

It is also worth encouraging the child to develop touch typing, as it is easier for them than having to concentrate on handwriting. Make sure that a computer is supplied during an exam at school or university so that he or she is not disadvantaged because of this.

Dyslexia can present problems when learning to drive, particularly during the theory test or if asked to read a number-plate during the practical test. The theory test has the option for dyslexic candidates to listen to the test being read in English or Welsh through a headset. Dyslexic candidates can also apply to have up to double the standard 57 minutes.

Before the practical test, it would be worth asking your optician for a letter confirming that you have good eyesight, in case you fail to read a number-plate. It may also be worth asking if you can read a number-plate with a yellow background. Also helpful could be requesting that the examiner indicates left and right with hand gestures rather than verbal instructions, and tells you the exit number on a roundabout.

If you feel anxious about letting the examiner know that you are dyslexic, raise the matter with your instructor and ask them to let the examiner know.

Dyslexia can also affect a person's ability to master a musical instrument. Sight-reading music can be difficult, particularly as you may not be able to take your time over it as you could reading a book. Remembering instructions in lessons and organising all the equipment needed can also be problematic.

It is worth speaking to the music teacher about dyslexia and explaining your needs, and asking them to show you how to do things rather than telling you. Once again, physical memory is key. Listening to pieces of music can also be an alternative to sight-reading. Special allowances can be made during music exams, such as examiners pointing at the right place on a page if a student becomes lost during a piece of music, and pointing when giving right-hand/left-hand instructions.

The award-winning director Steven Spielberg (also a dyslexic!) once said about dyslexia on the Friends of Quinn website: "It is more common than you can imagine. You are not alone. And while you will have this the rest of your life, you can dart between the raindrops to get where you want to go and it will not hold you back."

Yes. Most certainly. You are not alone.

Meet the charity

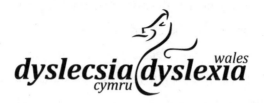

Dyslecsia Cymru / Wales Dyslexia could be of assistance if you have dyslexia.

Dyslexia affects between 10% and 15% of the population, but often there is a difficulty in getting recognition and support. The national dyslexia charity of Wales, Dyslecsia Cymru / Wales Dyslexia may be able to help you.

They offer:
→ Dyslexia screening in English and Welsh
→ Diagnostic assessments
→ Up-to-date assessments for application for additional funding for students studying in higher education
→ Programmes and workshops for remediation
→ Advice for dyslexic learners
→ Advice for dyslexic adults
→ Advice for parents of learners with (possible) dyslexia
→ Advice for educators
→ Advice for employers

The characteristics of dyslexia vary from person to person.

You may have some of the difficulties listed below, but answering 'yes' to any or all of these need not be evidence of dyslexia.

Do you, or someone you know, have difficulty with:
→ Reading
→ Writing
→ Spelling
→ Concentration / attention
→ Short-term memory
→ Organising / planning
→ Following instructions / directions

For more help and advice, please contact:
Freephone Bilingual Helpline 0808 1800 110
www.walesdyslexia.org.uk
REG CHARITY NUMBER: 1141416
Dyslecsia Cymru / Wales Dyslexia:
helping you reach your potential.

Other useful contact organisations and websites

Organisations and charities

The British Dyslexia Association offers information and support to people with dyslexia. It also campaigns for a dyslexia-friendly society.
www.bdadyslexia.org.uk
Helpline: 0333 405 4567

SNAP Cymru is a charity that offers information and support to families of children and young people who have special educational needs.
www.snapcymru.org
Helpline: 0845 120 3730

Dyslexia Action Wales provide support for people with dyslexia in Wales. Their services include one-to-one teaching, assessments, workplace consultations and awareness-raising sessions.
www.dyslexiaaction.wales

Resources

Crossbow Education sells teaching and learning aids for dyslexia.
www.crossboweducation.com
0845 269 7272

Teaching Reading Through Games (Trugs)
are literacy games to help children learn to read
(games are available in English and Welsh).
www.readsuccessfully.com
01752 663775

Technology

iansyst is an information technology
company that offers solutions, training and
consultancy for people with dyslexia.
www.iansyst.co.uk   01223 420101

Net Educational Systems sells educational software
that is suitable for children with dyslexia.
www.nessy.com   01179 239777

textHELP sells software that is suitable
for children with dyslexia.
www.texthelp.com/UK/Our-products/Fluency-Tutor
02894 4428105

Dyslexic.com sells software that is
suitable for people with dyslexia.
www.dyslexic.com   01223 420101

Claro Software sells software that
is suitable for dyslexics.
www.clarosoftware.com   01772 978096

Facts and figures on dyslexia
Source: Dyslexia Action

→ With at least 1 in 10 of the population estimated to have dyslexia, more than 6.3 million in the UK potentially have dyslexia

→ 1 in 5 children leave primary school with below the national expected levels in reading, writing and mathematics (formerly below national Level 4)

→ 1 in 10 children do not reach the expected national Level 4 in reading by the time they finish primary school (National Curriculum KS2)

→ 1 in 6 adults still only have the reading skills of an 11-year-old

→ Pupils with special educational needs (SEN) (with and without statements) account for 7 in 10 of all permanent exclusions

→ Pupils with SEN without statements are around ten times more likely to receive a permanent exclusion than pupils with no SEN; pupils with a statement of SEN are around six times more likely to receive a permanent exclusion

→ At secondary level, over a third of young people did not achieve the expected level of an A+ to C in English in 2014

→ There are approximately 955,000 young people (aged from 16 to 24) in the UK (August, 2014) not in Education, Employment or Training (NEET)

Congratulations on completing a 2018 Quick Read.

The Quick Reads project, with bite-sized books, is designed to get readers back into the swing of reading, and reading for pleasure. So we sincerely hope you enjoyed this book.

Got an opinion?

Your feedback can make this project better. Now you've read one of the Quick Reads series visit www.readingwales.org.uk or Twitter @quickreads2018 to post your feedback.

→ Why did you choose this book?

→ What did you like about it?

→ What do you think of the Quick Reads series?

→ Which Quick Reads would you like to see in the future?

What next?

Now that you've finished one Quick Read – got time for another?

Look out for the other title in the 2018 Quick Reads series – *No Place to Call Home* by Katey Pilling and Llinos Dafydd

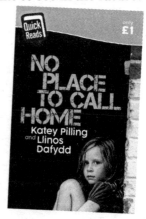